Mediterranean Diet

*The Complete Guide with Meal Plan and Recipes for Weight
Loss, Gain Energy and Burn Fat with Recipes
for Health lifestyle*

(Ultimate Mediterranean Recipes Cookbook)

Betty Leblanc

Published by Jason Thawne Publishing House

© Betty Leblanc

Mediterranean Diet: The Complete Guide with Meal Plan and Recipes for Weight Loss, Gain Energy and Burn Fat with Recipes for Health lifestyle

(Ultimate Mediterranean Recipes Cookbook)

All Rights Reserved

ISBN 978-1-989749-88-3

This document is geared towards providing exact and reliable information in regards to the topic and issue covered. The publication is sold with the idea that the publisher isn't required to render accounting, officially permitted, or otherwise, qualified services. If advice is necessary, legal or even professional, a practiced individual in the profession should be ordered.

From a Declaration of Principles which was accepted and approved equally by a Committee of the American Bar Association and a Committee of Publishers and Associations.

In no way is it legal to reproduce, duplicate, or even transmit any part of this document in either electronic means or in printed format. Recording of this publication is strictly prohibited and any storage of this document isn't allowed unless with proper written permission from the publisher. All rights reserved.

The information provided herein is stated to be truthful and consistent, in that any liability, in terms of inattention or otherwise, by any usage or abuse of any policies, processes, or directions contained within is the solitary and also utter responsibility of the recipient reader. Under no circumstances will any legal responsibility or blame be held against the publisher for any reparation, damages, or monetary loss due to the information herein, either directly or indirectly.

Respective authors own all copyrights not held by the publisher.

The information herein is offered for just informational purposes solely, and is universal as so. The presentation of the information is without contract or any type of guarantee assurance.

The trademarks that are used are without any consent, and also the publication of the trademark is without permission or backing by the trademark owner. All trademarks and brands within this book are for clarifying purposes only and are the owned by the owners themselves, not affiliated with this document.

TABLE OF CONTENTS

Part 1 1

Introduction 2

Chapter One: What Is The Mediterranean Diet In The First Place? 4

Chapter Two: The Healthy Benefits Of The Mediterranean Diet 8

Chapter Three: The Mediterranean Diet Food Pyramid ... 21

Tier One: Whole Grains 21

Tier Two: Vegetables, Legumes, Seeds, Fruits, Nuts And Beans 23

Tier Three: Olive Oil 27

Tier Four: Yogurt And Cheese 29

Tier One: Fish 31

Tier Two: Meat 33

Tier Three: Eggs 34

Tier Four: Poultry 35

Chapter Four: How The Mediterranean Diet Can Help With Weight Loss 36

What Are The General Principles Of This Diet? 43

Chapter Five: Delicious Mediterranean Recipes 48

Mediterranean Style Lettuce Wraps 48

Mediterranean Style Zucchini 50

Fresh Mozzarella And Tomato Skewers 51

Savory Tomato Soup 53

Grilled Balsamic Veggie Salad 55

Avocado And Spinach Salad 57

Cashew And Ginger Mushrooms 59

Savory Dijon And Lemon Honey Chicken 61

Delicious Quinoa Salad With Fresh Avocado And Dill 63

Hearty Zucchini And Red Pepper Stew.............................. 66

Delicious Avocado Tacos 68

Mediterranean Zucchini 70

Delicious Tomato Pasta 72

Strawberries Mixed With Balsamic Vinegar 74

Conclusion 76

Part 2... 78

Introduction 79

Chapter 1 All About The Mediterranean Diet.................... 80

THE MEDITERRANEAN DIET AND LIFESTYLE 80
WHAT CONSISTS THE MEDITERRANEAN DIET?............................. 82

Chapter 2 The Mediterranean Diet Food Pyramid And
Health Benefits.. 85

THE HEALTH BENEFITS OF THE MEDITERRANEAN DIET................... 86
The Risk Of Cardiovascular Disease Is Lessened 87
The Chance Of Having Type 2 Diabetes Is Lowered.......... 87
You Get To Lose Weight The Healthy Way 88
There Is A Reduced Chances Of Being At Risk Of Parkinson's
Disease 88
You Become Healthier - More Strength And Endurance.... 89

Chapter 3 Mediterranean Regional Ingredients 90

Chapter 4 Meal Plans And Recipes 98

BREAKFAST RECIPES 98

1. Berries And Mint Salad 98
2. Green And Red Fruits With Walnut Salad 98
3. Broccoli With Maple Syrup And Apple Cider Vinegar ... 100
4. Zucchini Salad Bruschetta 101
5. Spinach, Tomato, And Tofutti Cheese Frittata 102

LUNCH RECIPES 104

1. Quick And Easy Vegan Pesto Pasta 104
2. Spinach And Grape Tomatoes Salad 105
3. Coconut Curry Soup 106
4. Asparagus Rice 107
5. Baked Brussels Sprouts 108
6. Spinach-Stuffed Mushrooms 109
7. Mussels With Tomato Sauce 110
1. Stir-Fry Mixed Vegetables 112
2. Baked Tomatoes 113
3. Squash Soup 114
4. Corn And Spinach Rice 116
5. Broccoli Noodles 117
6. Zucchini Noodles 117
7. Carrot Noodles 118
8. Fish Stew With Tomatoes And Anchovies 119

DESSERT 120

1. Blue Cheese And Red Onion Marmalade 121
2. Spinach Flat Cakes 122
3. Broccoli Flat Cakes 123
4. Carrot Flat Cakes 124
5. Cranberry And Cherries Puddings 126
6. Apricots And Cherries Puddings 127
7. Swiss Chard Flat Cakes 130

Conclusion 131

About The Author 131

PART 1

INTRODUCTION

When people often hear the word "Mediterranean," most people often think about hour long feasts with foods such as pizza, lasagna, endless bottles of wine and lots of pasta. However, most of these dishes do not often fit the traditional style of Mediterranean cooking. Today most of the food that you can find in countries lining the Mediterranean Sea has transformed this cuisine into a much simpler and healthier line of cuisine than many people actually realize. Today this cuisine is more of a lifestyle than anything and it has been proven to contribute greatly to overall human health.

If you want to aim for a much slimmer and much healthier body, the Mediterranean diet is certainly the one that you want to follow. This science-backed "lifestyle approach" allows you to lose weight fast and safely without putting your precious health at risk. It is a way of life rather than a systemized diet plan. The foundation of this diet is eating basic yet healthy dishes influenced by the traditional cuisine of the countries surrounding the Mediterranean Sea.

In this book you will find a guide on how to live the Mediterranean lifestyle as well as a few delicious Mediterranean style recipes that are not only delicious, but that are healthy for you as well, and are easily maintained with your daily life.

I hope you enjoy this book and put these concepts of Mediterranean living to the best use to bring you the most abundant health and longevity for years to come!

CHAPTER ONE:
WHAT IS THE MEDITERRANEAN DIET IN THE FIRST PLACE?

The countries bordering the Mediterranean Sea have long impressed the Western world through breakthroughs in philosophy, culture, religion, politics, and science. But now, they are putting the whole world in fascination as science draws a direct connection between what is known as the "Mediterranean diet" and the lower risk and incidence of cancer, heart disease, diabetes, Alzheimer's disease, and obesity.

The name Mediterranean originates from the Latin word Mediterraneans, which means "in the middle of the land". The Mediterranean Sea is recognized for its important role in the flourishing of modern civilization. The sea joins the Black Sea and Sea of Marmara in the east, and the Atlantic Ocean in the west. Twenty-one coastal countries border the Sea: Albania, Algeria, Croatia, Egypt, France, Greece, Israel, Italy, Lebanon, Libya, Morocco, Spain, the State of Palestine, Syria, Tunisia, and Turkey. It served as an important path for merchants and travelers in the ancient times. It was, and probably still is, one of the primary sources of food of the civilizations that flourished around it.

The Mediterranean Sea is considered as a "biodiversity hotspot"— accommodating around 700 marine species, most of them indigenous. The Mediterranean region is a cradle of staples like figs, mandarins, hazelnuts, grapes, chickpeas, and olives. The region also credits its rocky, coastal terrain for healthy meat sources such as chicken, sheep, and lamb.

Ancel Keys, an American scientist, first brought Mediterranean diet in Pioppi, Italy 1945. However, it was not until the 1990s that the public and medical community fully embraced the Mediterranean diet's importance and benefits. Despite the name, the Mediterranean diet is not a complete representation of authentic Mediterranean cuisine. For instance, in Israel, Malta, and Egypt, use of olive oil is inessential; in Northern Italy, olive oil is for salad and cooked vegetables only. According to Dr. Walter Willett of Harvard University's School of Public Health, this diet is based on "food patterns typical of Crete, much of the rest of Greece, and southern Italy in the early 1960s."

The Mediterranean diet stresses the importance of daily consumption of whole-grain cereals, fresh fruits, vegetables and legumes; olive oil as the main source of fat; limited intake of dairy products; moderate consumption of meat, meat products, fish, fish products, poultry, and poultry products; and low to moderate consumption of wine. In addition, the Mediterranean diet highlights eating delightfully delicious dishes, which is the trademark of the Mediterranean cuisine. Just as important, it emphasizes the importance of regular physical activity and enjoying meals with family and friends, too. The United Nations Educational, Scientific and Cultural Organization (UNESCO) officially acknowledged the Mediterranean diet as a part of the cultural heritage of Greece, Italy, and Morocco in 2010.

Why Choose The Mediterranean Diet?

The Mediterranean diet is easy to adapt to your lifestyle. Unlike many diets that involve increasing your intake of certain vitamins and minerals, the Mediterranean diet is different in that it allows you to eat a wide variety of foods.

Also, the foods in the Mediterranean diet are foods that you already eat fairly regularly, so adapting to a Mediterranean way of eating would not involve any drastic changes.

CHAPTER TWO:
THE HEALTHY BENEFITS OF THE MEDITERRANEAN DIET

Improves Cardiovascular Health

Consumption of unhealthy fats such as polysaturated fat, saturated fat, and cholesterol are some of the factors that govern the causation of chronic conditions including hypertensive disorder and cardiovascular diseases. These fats, when ingested in unhealthy amounts, amass in the blood vessels. They also congest the blood vessels and impede the delivery of oxygen to the heart. As an effect, the cells in the heart will eventually die, causing myocardial infarction otherwise known as heart attack.

Hypertensive disorder is an alarming condition that kills many people around the world. This condition is so deadly that even a small rise from the normal blood pressure can kick-start a domino effect in the human body. For example, a rise in the normal blood pressure can cause the small capillaries to erupt, which in turn will cause migraine and, much worse, heart failure.

An increase in blood pressure causes the left ventricular hypertrophy to thicken which often results in less efficient pumping power. This leads to poor supply of blood and nutrients to the organs of the body, particularly during physical activities. To counterweigh reduced heart endurance, the heart's arteries stretch further in order to accommodate more blood volume. This keeps the blood flow normal for some time, but it puts the heart muscle strength at stake. Over the time, the heart muscle walls will weaken, will not be able to work as it should be, and will eventually collapse.

Following the Mediterranean diet can improve the cardiovascular fitness and blood circulation, especially of those people with concurrent cardiovascular conditions. According to a study published online February 25, 2013 in the New England Journal of Medicine, switching to Mediterranean diet can decrease risk to heart disease and strokes to about 3o percent. The study, which was conducted by Harvard School of Public Health Nutrition Experts, followed the lives of 7, 447 people with ages 55 to 80. These people had risk factors such as smoking habit, overweight, and diabetes. Some of them followed low fat diet, some of them Mediterranean. Investigators were surprised by how evident the findings were.

"Even the best available drugs, like statins, reduce heart disease by about 25%, which is in the same ballpark as the Mediterranean diet," according to Dr Willet, one of the professors who supervised the study. "But the statins increase the risk of diabetes, whereas this diet can help reduce the risk." In a separate study which was published online April 10, 2013 in the New England Journal of Medicine, researchers ranked the Mediterranean diet as the most likely dietary pattern for the prevention of cardiovascular events."

These benefits to the circulatory and cardiovascular system are because the Mediterranean diet is high in fiber, folate, healthy fats, and magnesium, but low in sodium and unhealthy fats like cholesterol, saturated fat, and polysaturated fat. Olive oil, the primary source of fat in Mediterranean diet, is one of the healthiest foods you can eat to improve heart health. It is teeming with monounsaturated fat, a healthy fat that improves cardiovascular fitness. Even better, olive oil prevents the oxidation of LDL particles, which plays a huge role in the development of heart disease.

Fiber from nuts, legumes, seeds, fruits, and vegetables has also been linked to significantly lower risk for cardiovascular complications. According to a study published in the Archive of Internal Medicine, eating at least 21 grams of fiber daily will result to 11 percent lower risk for cardiovascular disease and 12 percent lower risk for coronary heart disease.

Another nutrient that Mediterranean-style dishes have plenty of is magnesium, a nutrient found in most fiber-rich foods. This nutrient prevents heart cell degeneration by revitalizing heart cells, therefore improving cardiovascular endurance and lowering risk for heart attack. On the other hand, folate, found in legumes, nuts, and seeds effectively combats homocysteine, which is a byproduct that significantly increases the risk of peripheral heart disease, heart attack, and stroke.

Helps To Fight Off Type 2 Diabetes

The rate of people clinically diagnosed with diabetes has doubled in incidence globally within the past 30 years. Diabetes is a debilitating condition. People with this condition have difficulty having normal blood sugar because their bodies either lack the hormone insulin or do not use it correctly.

The good news is that people who follow Mediterranean diet experience significantly lower risks for type 2 diabetes. A research study, which followed the lives of Spanish men and women aged 55 to 80 for about four years, found that Mediterranean diet without the intervention of formal physical activity can significantly reduce the risk for diabetes. The study, which was published online in the Annals of Medicine, involved 3, 541 participants randomly assigned to three different groups: a Mediterranean diet with olive oil, a Mediterranean diet with mixed nuts, and a low-fat diet which served as the comparison.

Compared with the comparison diet group, the risk for diabetes was 40 percent lower with the group that followed the Mediterranean diet with olive oil, and 18 percent lower with the group that followed the Mediterranean diet with mixed nuts.

Dr. Ramón Estruch, one of the researchers in the study and an associate professor of Medicine at the University of Barcelona, noted, "The diet works by itself without considering physical activity or changes in weight, which were insignificant between groups."

Helps To Fight Off Obesity

Obesity is a prevalent medical condition, killing at least 2.8 million people worldwide every year. This condition is also correlated with many medical conditions, including coronary heart disease, stroke, gallstones, cancer, osteoarthritis, and diabetes mellitus.

People with body Mass Index (BMI) of 20 to 25 are overweight while those with BMI that exceeds 30 are obese.

Obese or overweight people have abnormally high fatty tissue, which causes abnormally high vascular resistance. High vascular resistance intensifies the workload of the heart and causes the organ to have trouble supplying blood to the body organs. Over the time, due to increased workload, the heart's muscle walls will thicken, will weaken, and will eventually collapse— a condition medically known as ventricular hypertrophy. In addition, obese people are more prone to heart attack (medically known as myocardial infarction) because abnormally high body fat destabilizes HDL to cholesterol ratio and LDL to cholesterol ratio, which are determining factors in the development of atherosclerosis (a condition wherein the arteries lose their elasticity).

Obese individuals also have higher risk for diabetes due to abnormal levels of body fat in the parts of the body, increased tolerance to glucose, and high levels of lipid and glucose.

The Framingham Study, a famous research study that lasted for 44 years proved that obesity and hypertensive disorder were two closely linked medical conditions. According to the study, 26 percent of men and 28 percent of women with hypertension got the disease because of obesity.

The Mediterranean diet can help fight obesity primarily because it is a formula for a healthy lifestyle rather than a whole list of foods to avoid. Moreover, unlike the typical American diet, the Mediterranean Diet allows dieters to consume good carbs as opposed to bad carbs, which can mostly be found in processed foods.

According to the study, which was published in the journal of the American College of Cardiology, Mediterranean diet reduces risk for obesity (the study also states that MD decreases risk for other debilitating conditions like diabetes and hypertensive disorder), because it significantly lowers the risk for metabolic syndrome by 50 percent.

Metabolic syndrome (an abnormality on energy storage and management) is one of the root causes of the development of the following medical conditions: obesity (particularly abdominal obesity), hypertensive disorder, cardiovascular diseases, and diabetes. A separate study, which was published September 6, 2012 in the online journal Wiley Online Library, states that Mediterranean diet's healthy food choices (fruits, vegetables, legumes, seeds, cereals, and olive oil) are helpful in the reduction of eventual weight gain and obesity among adults.

Helps To Preserve The Body's Endurance

The nutritional and health benefits that you can gain by following such diet can decrease the risk of the development of muscle and bone weakness and other symptoms of aging by 70 percent.

Helps To Reduce The Risk For Alzheimer's

A study, which was published November 21, 2006 in the online journal Neurology, reported that adherence to Mediterranean diet does not only lower risk for Alzheimer's disease (AD) but also impedes the eventual progress of the disease. In addition, according to the study, strict adherence to Mediterranean Diet resulted to lower incidence of death to AD, reflecting the possibility of dose-response effect.

Help To Reduce The Risk of Parkinson's

The Mediterranean Diet involves eating foods rich in anti-inflammatory agents such as fruits, vegetables, legumes, nuts, and olive oil. The olive oil, for example, has excellent amounts of anti-inflammatory agent called oleic acid. Anti-inflammatory compounds are proven to hamper the oxidation of cells, which is the main cause of Parkinson's disease. This benefit is further affirmed by a study, which was published 2008 in BMJ. According to it, strong adherence to the Mediterranean

Diet results to 13 percent reduction in the risk for Parkinson's disease.

Helps To Increase The Length of Your Life

The health benefits of the Mediterranean diet are tried and true. Just recently, a study, which was published in the Annals of Medicine, found that middle-aged women who adhered to the Mediterranean Diet were more likely to live beyond 70 without experiencing any debilitating medical conditions.

CHAPTER THREE: THE MEDITERRANEAN DIET FOOD PYRAMID

The Mediterranean diet food pyramid helps you make wise choices. Plus, it's simple to follow.

At the bottom of the pyramid are common staple foods that are to be consumed in large amounts and more frequently. Portion sizes and frequency decline as you go up the pyramid.

The pyramid is ordered in tiers that can help you plan your next meal. Each tier is categorized into either a daily, weekly or monthly group that provides an idea of how often certain foods should be eaten. Tier one is the lowest and widest tier on the pyramid and tier nine is the highest and smallest tier.

Daily Tiers

TIER ONE: WHOLE GRAINS

Whole grains are a source of "good carbs," vitamins and minerals, fiber and antioxidants that are to be consumed daily on the Mediterranean diet. These are the "fill you up" kinds of foods like rice and bread. In Italy, this tier often includes pasta.

Whole grains such as barley, bulgur, polenta, buckwheat, brown rice, farro, millet, whole wheat couscous, quinoa, wheatberries, breads, pasta and oats should be consumed at every meal in moderate amounts.

In the traditional Mediterranean diet, bread without butter or margarine was a key part of every meal. A typical meal would include pasta, polenta, potatoes or rice along with fresh vegetables and legumes and in other Mediterranean regions it was common to have bulgur and rice served with vegetables, chickpeas and various beans.

Nowadays the commercial processing of whole grains makes them less nutritious. Sugars and salts are added to packaged pasta and whole grain products to extend shelf life. Though they appear to be nutritious, the processing they undergo depletes them of most of their nutritional value and fiber.

It's best to buy wholegrain flour and make your own bread and pasta. That way you can determine how much salt and sugar is added. Whole grains are a good source of dietary fiber that prevents the absorption of unhealthy fat in the arteries.

8 servings of whole grains, non-refined cereal, brown rice, pasta and breads are suggested on the Mediterranean diet daily.

TIER TWO: VEGETABLES, LEGUMES, SEEDS, FRUITS, NUTS AND BEANS

Fruits and vegetables have always been consumed daily by people living in Mediterranean regions. The vegetables are normally cooked, raw and drizzled with olive oil.

In the traditional Mediterranean diet, plant foods accompanied every meal. Fresh vegetables, fruits, salads, nuts, seeds and olives were consumed regularly along with fresh herbs, garlic and onions. Seasonal use of local or homegrown vegetables would provide an abundance of antioxidants, dietary fiber and micronutrients naturally found in plant foods.

Many Mediterranean households typically have a vegetable garden and fruit trees in their yard. Even people that live in cities have window boxes in which they grow their own foods. For Mediterranean people, eating food in season, when nature intended, creates anticipation and allows them to live mindfully and enjoy the moment. The richness of this experience has been obscured by the American mega-marts availability of anything you want, whenever you want it.

In order to follow the Mediterranean tradition it is best to shop for local produce or grow your own vegetables and fruits. Seasonally fresh produce maximizes the nutrients that help fight heart disease.

Traditional Mediterranean diet vegetables include: carrots, cabbage, eggplant, fennel, artichokes, mushrooms, pumpkin, sweet potatoes, shallots, radishes, leeks, kale, lettuce, okra, peas, beets, broccoli, Brussels sprouts, peppers, scallions, rutabaga, arugula, celery, collard greens, dandelion greens, cucumbers, mache, eggplant, chicory, potatoes, spinach, turnips, zucchini, pumpkin, purslane, nettles, lemons, celeriac.

A variety of fresh plant foods should make up the bulk of your meals. Fruits in Mediterranean regions are normally eaten daily for dessert although having both fruits and vegetables as snacks throughout the day is encouraged.

Fruits common to Mediterranean tradition include: grapefruit, oranges, apricots, apples, oranges, pears, strawberries, peaches, avocados, cherries, figs, grapes, tomatoes, nectarines, olives, dates, melons, tangerines, pomegranates, clementines, melons.

The primary vegetarian sources of protein on the Mediterranean diet are beans and legumes. These include chickpeas, white beans, green beans, peas, lentils, butter beans, fava beans, cannellini beans, kidney beans and split peas.

Nuts, seeds and legumes that are common in the traditional Mediterranean diet include: walnuts, almonds, cashews, hazelnuts, sesame seeds, pistachios and pine nuts.

Herbs and spices are also traditionally used in Mediterranean cuisine to replace salt and increase flavor. They have an intriguing place in Mediterranean culture as both medicine and food. Salt is allowed on the Mediterranean diet but in smaller quantities than you might be used to.

Common herbs and spices include garlic, basil, oregano, parsley, thyme, mint, cloves, cumin, sage, pepper, fennel, bay leaf, anise, savory, rosemary, tarragon, lavender, marjoram, chilies, zatar, sumac and pul biber.

Garlic was primarily responsible for maintaining good blood pressure levels in Mediterranean countries during the Seven Country Study due to its ability to dilate the blood vessels.

6 servings of vegetables a day are suggested as well as 3 servings of fruit daily.

TIER THREE: OLIVE OIL

Ever since the Greek goddess Athena gave the olive tree to the Athenians, olive oil and olives has been an integral part of the diet of Greeks and Mediterranean people.

The health benefits of olive oil are massive, and research reveals more health benefits every day. Olive oil is at the core of the Mediterranean diet and is responsible for much of the

Mediterranean diets health promoting effects.

Olive oil is the primary source of fat on the Mediterranean diet and replaces animal fats. It contains numerous bioactive and antioxidant components like phytosterols, vitamin E and polyphenols.

Olive oil is one of the few culinary oils that have a fat content that is made up of 75% oleic acid. Oleic acid is a monounsaturated, omega-9 fatty acid that helps decrease blood pressure, protect cell membranes from free radicals and alleviate Type 2 diabetes. It also helps burn fat and has a number of other health benefits.

The combination of olive oil along with leafy salads and vegetables is what is believed to give the Mediterranean diet its health advantage. The unsaturated fat in the olive oil paired with the nitrogen compounds in the greens and vegetables produce a new group of compounds called nitro fatty acids. Nitro fatty acids cause reactions that result in the dilation of blood vessels that in turn lower blood pressure.

In buying olive oil it is important to choose good quality, fresh olive oil in order to receive the best health benefits that olive oil has to offer. Look for green oil in a dark bottle. It will be expensive but fine quality extra virgin olive oil is well worth the price. People in Italy often have their own olive grove and make their own fresh, stone pressed olive oil every year. Olives are normally eaten whole and are used in the Mediterranean region for cooking and flavoring. Greek-style black ripe olives contain natural antioxidants that help reduce inflammation, fight cancer, maintain bone mass and promote heart health.

Olives are actually a fruit. They are high in good fats, particularly monounsaturated fats and they are a rich nutritious source of 25 phytonutrients. They contain no cholesterol and they are low in carbs and Sodium.

TIER FOUR: YOGURT AND CHEESE

Dairy products are an important part of the Mediterranean diet. They are listed higher up on the Mediterranean pyramid so they are not to be consumed in the same amounts as the whole grain, vegetable, fruit and nut categories. They are however to be consumed daily – just in smaller amounts.

In the traditional Mediterranean diet, refrigeration was often lacking and the climate was normally hot, so milk was preserved and eaten as yogurt and cheese. Grating a small amount of cheese over a pasta dish was very typical.

If you think of the beautiful cheeses of France, Italy and Spain you can see why dairy products have become indicative of Mediterranean cuisine . The biggest and most important difference to keep in mind is that Mediterranean dairy products are not made from cow's milk; rather they are made from sheep, buffalo or goats milk.

Some examples of Mediterranean cheeses would be delicious feta cheeses made from goat's milk or Italy's famous mozzarella cheese made from buffalo or sheep's milk. Sheep and goat's milk have a lower amount of animal fat in them. Animal fat is known to clog arteries and damage our cardiovascular health.

Tzatziki is an example of a typical way that Greeks would use yogurt. Yogurt can also be used as part of a pasta sauce or as sour cream. Greek yogurt is different from regular yogurt in that it is extensively strained to remove the liquid lactose sugar and whey. This gives Greek yogurt its thick consistency. Greek yogurt can also contain double the protein of regular yogurt while cutting sugar content in half.

Weekly Tiers
TIER ONE: FISH

Fish is the most common type of meat eaten on the Mediterranean diet and is typically consumed two to three times a week up to five or six times (including a variety of seafood as well as fish).

Mediterranean fish markets daily display the catch of the day in order to provide their customers with the freshest fish available. To stay true to the Mediterranean tradition it is best to buy your fish from your local fishmonger rather than packaged supermarket fish. That way you will be getting the freshest fish that you can.

Oily fish that are packed with protein and omega-3 oils are an important part of the Mediterranean diet. These oils are consumed in dangerously low amounts in North America and Britain. Omegas are certain kinds of polyunsaturated fatty acids. Omega-3's are often called omega-3 essential fatty acids because the body needs them but can't make them. The only way of getting omega-3 fatty acids is by consuming them.

Two crucial types of omega-3's are EPA and DHA. These omega-3's are mostly found in certain kinds of fish. ALA is another kind of omega-3 oil that can be found in nuts and seeds. Omega-3's are crucial to the normal functioning of our bodies. Omega-3 fatty acids benefit your heart, regulate cholesterol triglyceride levels, prevent and alleviate joint pain and stiffness, fight depression, help our circulatory systems and prevent Alzheimer's and dementia.

Fish and seafood common to the area that contain omega-3' s are salmon (wild contains more than farmed), tuna, sardines, oysters, shrimp, crab, clams, mussels, sea bass, eel, flounder, lobster, abalone, tilapia, squid, octopus, cockles and whelk.

TIER TWO: MEAT

At the very top of the pyramid is red meat. Red meat should be limited to no more than four times a month. The positive health findings of the research done on the dietary patterns of the people of Crete, Greece, Spain and Italy in the 1950' s were at a point when poverty was high and farming was a way of life.

People had to rely on their livestock for labor so to consider using them as sustenance was normally out of the question. That is why there was very little red meat consumption at that time. Eating lean cuts of red meat in small amounts a few times a month is fine. Red meat common to the area include: lamb, beef, goat, guinea fowl, port, mutton and duck.

1-4 servings of red meat are suggested per month.

TIER THREE: EGGS

The Mediterranean diet recommends eating eggs at least a couple times a week to a maximum of four times a week. An egg is a complete meal in itself. It contains many of the necessary nutrients that the body needs. It does however have a higher cholesterol level and that is why it is not recommended that eggs be consumed daily.

Buy free range, organic eggs. You might even want to consider having a few chickens of your own in order to ensure that you are getting good quality eggs. Keeping chickens is inexpensive and doesn't take up much space. Chicken, quail and duck eggs are all common to Mediterranean cooking.

2-4 eggs a week are suggested per week.

TIER FOUR: POULTRY

Poultry is the second most common meat eaten on the Mediterranean diet. It is an excellent source of protein and can be eaten two to four times a week. In rural areas of the Mediterranean it is typical for people to have their own chickens in order to ensure freshness and make sure that their meat is not laden with chemicals.

In keeping with true Mediterranean tradition, buy free range, organic chicken.

2-4 servings of poultry are suggested per week.

CHAPTER FOUR:
HOW THE MEDITERRANEAN DIET CAN HELP WITH WEIGHT LOSS

For the past several years, the Mediterranean Diet has been receiving praises as one of the best diet plans to follow if you want to lose excess weight. In fact, it is among the diet plans with a high rate of adherence. Dietitians, dieters, nutritionists, and the majority of the medical community all agree that the Mediterranean Diet is effective not only for achieving better health but also for achieving a slimmer body figure.

One thing that makes Mediterranean Diet standout is the fact that it does not center on a single nutritional group. It is a healthy way of eating for life and not just a one-time fix to your health and weight. Even better, the components of the Mediterranean Diet are available to the public, meaning everyone wanting to have better health and weight can easily follow the Mediterranean Diet. If you are not convinced yet, below are the main reasons why the Mediterranean Diet is the thing to follow for healthier, slimmer body. You know it's time for the big switch.

The Mediterranean Diet Is A Great Diet To Follow

The Mediterranean Diet represents the true meaning of a balanced diet. While many fad diets out there put your health at risk for the sake of slimmer body figure, the Mediterranean Diet doesn't. The Mediterranean diet's approach leaves the body with essential nutrients and the palate with the delightfulness of Mediterranean-style cuisine.

The adverse effect of a diet shift is something you should not be worried about. The body can easily adjust to this new eating habit because the food choices that Mediterranean Diet introduces are nothing too unfamiliar and are all part of the basic food groups. Please be reminded, though, that withdrawal symptoms might still occur especially if you were dependent to sugary, salty, and fatty foods for years.

This Diet Helps To Put A Stop To Unhealthy Eating Habits

One of the main causes of obesity is unhealthy eating behavior. Amazingly, the Mediterranean diet can suppress unhealthy eating habits such as food bingeing and craving. Mediterranean-style dishes offer lots of fiber and protein, which are integral in suppressing unhealthy eating behaviors.

Unhealthy eating behaviors are because of the effects of sugary and fatty foods in the brain's neuroadaptive response, which is the same mechanism affected when one uses hard drugs. The more you consume sugar, the more problematic your unhealthy eating behaviors would be. Fiber is essential for suppressing unhealthy eating behaviors because it provides satiety, which is the state of being contented on what you eat. Medical experts believe that satiety plays a big role in overcoming abnormal eating behaviors and metabolic syndrome. In addition, fiber contains digestive enzymes, which cure inflammations along the digestive tract lining. An impaired digestive tract lining often causes craving for foods.

The abundance of protein in Mediterranean dishes provides energy that last for hours. One of the root causes of sugar addiction is shortage of body energy. People who developed sugar addiction tended to look for a quick way to boost their energy level. Sugar boosts energy in a few minutes time, but it also spikes insulin level, which immediately makes you hungry and tired— craving for more sugar knowing that it's a great energy source. Even worse, sugar spikes levels of hormone serotonin, which is a part of the brain's neurodaptive response. An increased serotonin level intensifies the desire to consume more sweets. Unlike sugar, protein carries carbohydrates in a way that doesn't spike the levels of insulin, blood sugar and serotonin, which are the governing factors of sugar addiction.

In addition, the Mediterranean Diet provides a wide variety of dishes. Another determining factor in the development of unhealthy eating behaviors is "food boredom", which occurs when the serotonin levels in the brain go low. Eating sugary and fatty foods do not lower serotonin levels, which explain why consuming such foods lead to food addiction. It is not normal that people who develop unhealthy eating behaviors are those that are tired and bored of what they eat because they're given very limited food choices. By providing a wide variety of delightful Mediterranean-style dishes, followers of the Mediterranean Diet would never again look for sugary and fatty foods to satisfy themselves.

The Mediterranean Diet Helps To Provide Healthy Carbohydrates

Many diet programs teach their dieters to lower consumption of carbs as much as possible. However, calories are essential for the body to thrive. At first, getting rid of carbs might sound a good idea. By consuming fewer calories, you will lose weight fast! However, blaming an entire food group for problems related to weight loss is a false approach to health and eating.

You must know that there are good and bad sources of carbohydrates. The good sources include unprocessed or natural and dietary foods such as legumes, whole grain foods, and vegetables. The bad sources , on the other hand, include practically all processed products like packaged goods, sodas, ready-to eat foods, and white flour-based foods (donuts, crackers, pasta, chips, and white bread).

Excluding carbs from the diet is very dangerous. Super low carbs in the body are not only equal to super low body fat, but also to super low muscle mass. As you probably already know, muscles are of utmost importance for rapid fat burning. An increased physical activity is equal to lower body fat. By losing your muscles, you won't be able to take advantage of their contribution to weight loss. Even then, who wishes to lose their muscles? In addition, an abrupt and huge body fat loss, which can only be possible by depriving yourself of carbs , can result to a rush of free radicals in the body. Overwhelming amount of free radicals can be shocking to the body. It causes kidney failure, brain damage, and blood toxicity.

How To Follow The Mediterranean Diet

The word "Mediterranean" only refers to the roots of the diet instead of the habit of eating Greek, Italian, or Egyptian cuisines. This diet pattern entails a wide variety of dietary foods shown to improve health and maintain body weight. In addition, the Mediterranean Diet allows dieters to have multiple sources of principal nutrients. For instance, through Mediterranean diet you get to eat wide variety of fruits, which allows you to have access to various essential nutrients.

WHAT ARE THE GENERAL PRINCIPLES OF THIS DIET?

Followers of the Mediterranean diet must know that the definitive rule in this is to have a healthy yet appetizingly satisfying eating habit over the long term. It is not about strictly following a formal diet plan nor is it about strictly avoiding certain foods. The Mediterranean diet heavily relies on lean protein meat, fruits and veggies, whole grain produce, legumes, and healthy fats. Below are the Mediterranean diet's general principles:

1. Increase Your Consumption of Veggies and Fruit

Vegetables and fruits are a great source of primary nutrients such as Vitamin C, Vitamin A, Potassium, Calcium, Magnesium, folate, and fiber. These foods also help reduce likelihood of heart disease, diabetes, stroke, several types of cancer, and help fight against the two most common reasons of vision loss, cataract and macular degeneration.

2. Increase Consumption of Wholegrain Foods

Grains are one of the hallmarks of Mediterranean diet. They are a staple in the traditional cuisines of the lands bordering the Mediterranean Sea. Generally, as long as they are whole, there is no harm on eating grains daily. Wholegrain produce is high in fiber, protein, minerals, complex carbs, and anti-inflammatory compounds. These foods reduce risk of irritable bowel problems, some types of cancer, diabetes, heart disease and obesity, improves memory, improves digestion and metabolism, balances blood sugar and lowers bad fat in the blood. Unlike their refined version, whole grains have prominently lower amounts of cholesterol, saturated fat, calories, and polysaturated fat, which make them highly recommended for weight and health management.

3. Enjoy Seafood Weekly

Unsurprisingly, seafood is an essential part of Mediterranean cuisines. The Mediterranean Sea is abundant in tasty , healthy , and inexpensive seafood like anchovies, sardines, tuna, mackerel and squid— making these foods a fundamental part of the Mediterranean diet. Seafood is high in Vitamin A, Vitamin D, protein, and essential minerals. Most fish have high amounts of omega 3 fatty acids as well, which further makes them a must-eat for your heart health.

4. Consume More Legumes and Nuts

Legumes, seeds, and nuts are staples of various Mediterranean cuisines, thanks to their tangy yet rich flavor. However, these foods are a must not only because they satisfy the palate, but also because of their significant contribution to weight and overall health. These foods are high in fiber, protein , Vitamin C, and Vitamin B. Just like fruits, they also deliver complex carbohydrates. Such foods reduce risk for a whole host of diseases including heart disease, stroke, hypertension, diabetes, obesity and arthritis. These also sharpens memory, improves digestion, and metabolism. However, nuts have considerably high amounts of calories, which is why they must be limited in small portions or three to five one-ounce servings a week.

CHAPTER FIVE:
DELICIOUS MEDITERRANEAN RECIPES

MEDITERRANEAN STYLE LETTUCE WRAPS

This dish is packed with delicious veggies, crunchy vegetables and fresh ginger. This dish is not only very colorful, but it tastes great as well.

Total Prep Time: **22 Minutes**

Serves: 8 Wraps

Ingredients:

- 2 tsp. of Canola Oil
- 1 Clove of Garlic, Minced
- 2 Tbsp. of Hoisin Sauce
- 1 Pinch of Red Chili Peppers, Dried
- 2 tsp. of Gingerroot, Grated Finely
- ½ tsp. of Sesame Oil

- A few Leaves of Lettuce
- 1/3 Cup of Coriander, Fresh and Chopped Finely
- 1/3 Cup of Green Onion, Chopped Finely
- ½ Cup of Cucumber, Diced Into Thin Pieces
- ½ Cup of Carrot, Shredded
- ½ Cup of Red Pepper, Sweet and Diced Into Small Pieces

Directions:

1. In a large sized non-stick skillet, heat up some oil over low to medium heat. Add in your garlic and ginger root and allow to cook for the next 2 minutes or until they become soft and light brown in color.

2. Next stir in your sesame oil and hoisin sauce. Add in your chili peppers and stir until well mixed. Reduce your heat to the lowest setting and cook for the next 5 minutes.

3. Remove from heat and lay out your lettuce wraps on a flat surface. Take about 3 Tbsp. of your vegetable filling onto each leaf of lettuce and wrap like a burrito. Enjoy.

MEDITERRANEAN STYLE ZUCCHINI

If you are a fan of Mediterranean cuisine then you are going to love this recipe. Feel free to serve this dish over a side of rice or nutritious egg noodles to make the perfect dinner meal.

Total Prep Time: **60 Minutes**

Serves: 6

Ingredients:

- 3 Cloves of Garlic, Crushed and Minced
- 2 Cups of Water

- 3 Tbsp. of Olive Oil
- 1 Red Bell Pepper, Finely Chopped
- 1 Onion, Large In Size and Chopped Finely
- 1 Cup of White Rice, Long Grain
- Dash of Salt and Pepper For Taste
- 1, 14 Ounce Can of Tomatoes, Peeled and Chopped Finely
- 3 Cups of Zucchini, Chopped Into Small Pieces
- ½ tsp. of Oregano, Dried
- 1, 15 Ounce Can of Cannellini Beans, Drained and Rinsed

Directions:

FRESH MOZZARELLA AND TOMATO SKEWERS

This is one of the fastest appetizer recipes that you will ever make. They look beautiful and are packed full of fresh taste, giving you a dish that you won't soon forget. While it may be a simple recipe to make, this is a dish that will certainly shine at your dinner table.

Total Prep Time: **20 Minutes**

Makes: 6 Servings

Ingredients

- 2 Cups of Tomatoes, Cherry and Fresh
- 6 Ounces of Mozzarella, Fresh and Cut Into Small Cubes or Balls
- 6 Leaves of Basil, Fresh
- Dash of Salt and Pepper For Taste
- 2 Tbsp. of Olive Oil
- A Handful of Skewers or Toothpicks, Wooden

Directions:

1. Gently place your fresh mozzarella and tomatoes onto your wooden skewers or toothpicks.

2. Then garnish your skewers with your basil leaves and dash of salt and pepper. Place them onto a serving plate and drizzle with a touch of olive oil. Serve immediately and enjoy.

SAVORY TOMATO SOUP

While this tomato soup looks anything but different when you first look at it, but the moment that you taste it for the first time you will immediately taste all of those wonderful Mediterranean flavors that will send your taste buds straight to heaven. There is no need to add anything more to this dish as it already has everything you are looking for.

Total Prep Time: **45 Minutes**

Makes: 6 Servings

Ingredients:

- 2 Tbsp. of Olive Oil
- 1 Shallot, Medium In Size and Chopped Finely
- 2 Cloves of Garlic, Finely Chopped
- 12 Inches of Grass Stalk, Lemon and Crushed
- 4 Tomatoes, Heirloom, Peeled and Chopped Finely
- 1 tsp. of Ginger, Grated
- Dash of Salt and Pepper
- 3 Cups of Vegetable Stock
- 1 tsp. of Hot Sauce, Your Favorite Brand

Directions:

1. Using a large sized soup pot, heat up your olive oil over medium to high heat and then add in your minced garlic and chopped shallot. Sauté these for the next 2 minutes or until fragrant.

2. Then add in the rest of your ingredients and allow the soup to cook for the next 20 to 25 minutes.

3. Remove from heat and toss out your lemongrass stalk. Pour your soup into a blender and puree your soup until it reaches the desired consistency that you want.

4. Pour your soup into serving bowls and serve either warm or chilled. Enjoy.

GRILLED BALSAMIC VEGGIE SALAD

If you are looking for a salad recipe that will enhance the natural flavor and sweetness of your veggies, this is the salad recipe for you. While still preserving all of the important nutrients this recipe will bring you a dish that tastes smoky and is absolutely delicious.

Total Prep Time: **35 Minutes**

Makes: 6 Servings

Ingredients:

- 1 Zucchini, Fresh and Sliced Thinly
- 1 Eggplant, Fresh, Peeled and Sliced Thinly
- 2 Tomatoes, Ripe and Sliced Finely
- 1 Carrot, Fresh and Cut Lengthwise Very Finely
- 1 Onion, Red In Color and Sliced Finely
- 2 Yellow Bell Pepper, Fresh, Cored and Sliced Into Quarters
- 2 Tbsp. of Olive Oil

- ¼ Cup of Vinegar, Balsamic
- Dash of Salt and Pepper For Taste
- 4 Cloves of Garlic, Chopped Finely

Directions:

1. Using a medium sized saucepan, heat it over high heat and place all of your vegetables into it, one by one.

2. Sauté your veggies until they are brown on each side and then remove from heat. Place them into a medium sized mixing bowl.

3. Using a separate bowl mix up your balsamic vinegar, dash of salt and pepper for taste, olive oil and garlic together until evenly combined.

4. Pour your new dressing over your grilled veggies and serve immediately. Enjoy.

AVOCADO AND SPINACH SALAD

The best part about this salad can be either the rich flavor of the poppy seeds that you use for the dressing or the creamy texture of the avocado. The contrast between these two ingredients helps make this a dish that is both filling and delicious.

Total Prep Time: **20 Minutes**

Makes: 6 Servings

Ingredients:

- 2 Tbsp. of Almonds, Sliced
- 1 Pound of Spinach, Baby
- 1 Avocado, Ripe, peeled and Sliced
- 1 Tbsp. of Poppy Seeds
- ½ of A Lemon, juiced
- 1 tsp. of Honey
- 1 tsp. of Lemon Zest, Fresh
- 1 Tbsp. of Olive Oil

- Dash of Salt and Pepper For Taste
- 1 tsp. of Vinegar, Apple Cider

Directions:

1. In a salad bowl combine your avocado, spinach and almonds until gently mixed together.

2. In a small sized mixing bowl combine the rest of your ingredients together to make your dressing. Stir together until thoroughly mixed.

3. Drizzle your dressing over your salad and serve while as fresh as possible.

CASHEW AND GINGER MUSHROOMS

This is another great side dish that you can make and that will go perfect with nearly any Whole 30 meal that you make.

Total Prep Time: 20 Minutes
Makes: 4 Servings

Ingredients:

- 1 Pound of Mushrooms, Rinsed and Then Dried Thoroughly
- 2 tsp. of Ginger, Grated
- ½ Cup of Cashews, Pieces
- 2 Tbsp. of Coconut Aminos
- 1 Tbsp + 1 tsp. of Coconut Oil, Divided

Directions:

1. Using a large non-stick skillet, heat up your 1 tsp. of Coconut Oil over low to medium heat. Sauté your cashew pieces in the skillet until they turn golden brown in color. This should take about 1 to 2 minutes. Set aside for later use.

2. Using the same pan heat up your 1 Tbsp. of Coconut Oil low the same heat and place your mushrooms into it. Allow your mushrooms to cook for about 2 minutes or until the bottoms begin to turn golden brown in color. Stir and then leave to cook for 8 minutes or until the mushrooms become tender.

3. Add in your coconut aminos and grate ginger to your skillet and reduce the heat to low. Stir to thoroughly combine the ingredient and allow to cook for 1 minute untouched.

4. Stir in your cashews last and allow the entire dish to heat thoroughly before serving.

SAVORY DIJON AND LEMON HONEY CHICKEN

For a savory meal that is simply to cook, this is the dish for you. Everything that you need to compliment this dish is included and it will surely satisfy all of your taste buds.

Total Prep Time: 6 to 8 Hours and 20 Minutes
Makes: 10 Plates

Ingredients:

- 2 Large Slices of Chicken Breasts, Skinless and Boneless
- 10 Cloves of Garlic, Freshly Peeled and sliced Thinly
- 15 Red Potatoes, Cut Into Quarters
- 2 Cups of Chicken Broth, Reduced Sodium
- 1 tsp. of Salt
- 2 Tbsp. of Dijon Mustard
- 1 Medium Sized Lemon, Seeds Removed and Sliced Into Thin Pieces
- 2 Tbsp. of Honey
- 2 Cups of Onions, Pearled and The Ends Trimmed Off
- ½ Cup of French Green Beans
- Dash of Pepper for Taste
- ¼ Cup of Fresh Parsley, Finely Chopped
- 2 Tbsp. of Fresh Thyme, Chopped Finely

Directions

1. Turn your crock pot on to the setting that you desire and place your chicken breasts, lemon, chicken broth, salt, pepper, potatoes, pearl onions, garlic and French green beans into it.

2. Cover and cook for either 6 to 8 hours on the lowest setting or cook for 3 to 4 hours on the highest setting.

3. Once it has finished cooking remove both the chicken breasts and the lemon slices. Slice your chicken into fine and thin slices and place them back into the crock-pot. Next stir in your Dijon Mustard and honey then add in the thyme and parsley, stirring as you do so. Season with the desired amount of salt and Pepper and serve. Enjoy.

DELICIOUS QUINOA SALAD WITH FRESH AVOCADO AND DILL

What lunch is completely without a salad. If you haven't gotten the chance to try Quinoa yet, this recipe will help you fall in love with it. Feel free to be creative as you want with this recipe and add in whatever additional vegan friendly ingredients that you want.

Total Prep Time: **30 Minutes**

Serves: 4 to 6

Ingredients:

- 1 Cup of Quinoa, Golden
- 1 Shallot, Large In Size and Chopped Finely
- 1 ¾ Cups of Vegetable Broth
- 8 Radishes, Small In Size and Chopped Finely
- 2/3 Cups of Dill, Stems Gone
- 3 Tbsp. of Olive Oil, Extra Virgin
- ½ Tbsp. of Vinegar, Balsamic
- ½ Cup of Almonds, Sliced Finely
- ½ Cup of Dates, Chopped Roughly

- ½ Lemon, Fresh and Used From Juice and Zest
- 1/3 of a Cucumber, Sliced Thinly
- Dash of Salt and Pepper For Taste
- 1 Avocado, Ripe and Cut Into Small Chunks

Directions:

1. Rinse your quinoa while using a fine mesh strainer for at least 2 to 3 minutes, making sure to rub the quinoa vigorously while you are doing it.

2. In a medium sized saucepan heat up your extra virgin olive oil and cook your quinoa in the oil for about 1 to 2 minutes. Then pour in your vegetable broth and allow to come to a boil. Once it does turn the heat down to the lowest setting and allow to cook for about 15 minutes. After 15 minutes remove from heat and allow to sit for 5 minutes.

3. Drain your quinoa and place into a bowl to allow to cool completely.

4. Place your remaining ingredients into a small sized mixing bowl and toss until all of the ingredients are thoroughly combined. Toss in your quinoa and stir until well mixed.

5. Serve into a salad bowl and enjoy immediately.

HEARTY ZUCCHINI AND RED PEPPER STEW

This dish will satisfy you unlike any other Mediterranean style dish that you come across. It is hearty and savory, making this a dish that you will want to make all of the time.

Total Prep Time: 1 Hour and 20 Minutes
Serves: 4 Servings

Ingredients:

- ¼ Cup of Olive Oil
- ½ Cup of Rice, Basmati

- 1 Eggplant, Sliced Into 1 Inch Cubes
- 5 Cloves of Garlic, Chopped Finely
- 3 Tomatoes, Fresh and Diced Into Small Pieces
- 1 Cup of Onions, Chopped Finely
- 1 Red Bell pepper, Chopped Into Small Pieces
- 1 ½ Cups of Water, Warm
- ¼ tsp. of Red Pepper Flakes
- ¼ Cup of Basil, Fresh
- ½ tsp. of Salt and Pepper For Taste
- ¼ Cup of Parsley, Fresh and Chopped Finely
- 1 Sprig of Rosemary, Fresh and Chopped
- 1 Cup of Wine, Marsala

Directions:

1. Place your eggplant into a medium sized colander and sprinkle with your dash of salt and pepper. Slice up your eggplant and sauté in a pan with some oil until it is slightly brown in color. Then stir in your onion and sauté until the onions are translucent. Next add in your garlic and sauté with your eggplant and onion for about 2 to 3 minutes.

2. Then stir in your rice, tomatoes, water, red pepper flakes, some additional salt, pepper, zucchini and red bell pepper. Make sure your cook your mixture over medium heat until it reaches a nice rolling boil and then reduce the heat. Allow to simmer for about 45 minutes or until all of your vegetables are tender.

3. Remove from heat and stir in your rosemary, basil and parsley until thoroughly combined. Serve while still piping hot.

DELICIOUS AVOCADO TACOS

These tacos are simple and easy to make and taste amazing as well. You will want to make this dish all of the time.

Total Prep Time: **25 Minutes**

Serves: 6

Ingredients:

- ¼ Cup of Onions, Diced Into Small Pieces
- 3 Avocados, Peeled, Pitted and Mashed Into A Smooth Consistency
- ¼ tsp. of Garlic Salt
- Dash of Jalapeno Pepper Sauce, For Taste
- 12 Corn Tortillas
- Some Fresh Leaves of Cilantro, Chopped Finely

Directions:

1. Preheat your oven to 325 degrees.
2. While your oven heats up, take out a medium sized mixing bowl. In the bowl

mix up your garlic salt, avocado and onions until it reaches a smooth consistency.

3. Then arrange your tortillas on a greased baking sheet and place into your oven for 2 to 5 minutes so that they are heated through. Then spread your avocado mixture onto your tortillas and garnish with some fresh cilantro and jalapeno pepper sauce. Serve immediately.

MEDITERRANEAN ZUCCHINI

If you are a fan of Mediterranean cuisine then you are going to love this recipe. Feel free to serve this dish over a side of rice or nutritious egg noodles to make the perfect dinner meal.

Total Prep Time: **60 Minutes**

Serves: 6

Ingredients:

- 3 Cloves of Garlic, Crushed and Minced
- 2 Cups of Water
- 3 Tbsp. of Olive Oil
- 1 Red Bell Pepper, Finely Chopped
- 1 Onion, Large In Size and Chopped Finely
- 1 Cup of White Rice, Long Grain
- Dash of Salt and Pepper For Taste
- 1, 14 Ounce Can of Tomatoes, Peeled and Chopped Finely
- 3 Cups of Zucchini, Chopped Into Small Pieces
- ½ tsp. of Oregano, Dried
- 1, 15 Ounce Can of Cannellini Beans, Drained and Rinsed

Directions:

1. In a medium sized saucepan, bring some water oven medium heat and stir in your rice. Allow to simmer for about 20 minutes until it is fully cooked.

2. In another saucepan, heat up some oil over low to medium heat. Stir in your garlic, onion and red bell pepper. Stir consistently until the mixture becomes fully tender. Mix in your tomatoes and zucchini next. Season with some salt, pepper and oregano and cover your skillet. Reduce your heat and allow to simmer for the next 20 minutes, making sure to stir as frequently as possible.

3. Then stir in your bean to your mixture and let cook for an additional 10 minutes. Once done serve over your cooked rice and enjoy.

DELICIOUS TOMATO PASTA

This is an extremely simple recipe to make and you will want to make it as frequently as possible. Feel free to use whatever kind of pasta that you like.

Total Prep Time: **22 Minutes**

Serves: 2

Ingredients:

- 1 Tomato, Medium In Size and Coarsely Chopped
- 1 Clove of Garlic, Coarsely Chopped
- Dash of Salt and Pepper For Taste
- 1 tsp. of Basil, Dried
- 1 Tbsp. of Olive Oil
- 1 Package of Pasta of Your Choice, Dried

Directions:

1. Cook your pasta thoroughly in a large pot of boiling water. Cook until pasta is al dente, drain and set aside to use later.

2. In a small mixing bowl combine your tomatoes, basil, olive oil and salt. Toss until all of the ingredients are thoroughly mixed. Pour over your cooked pasta and serve. Enjoy.

STRAWBERRIES MIXED WITH BALSAMIC VINEGAR

When you mix strawberries with some balsamic vinegar, you will help bring out the strawberries true flavor. Feel free to serve this dish with some pound cake or with some ice cream.

Total Prep Time: 1 Hour and 10 Minutes
Serves: 6

Ingredients:

- 16 Ounces of Strawberries, Fresh and Cut In Half

- 2 Tbsp. of Vinegar, Balsamic
- ¼ tsp of Black Pepper For Taste
- ¼ Cup of Sugar, White

Directions:

1. Place your strawberries into a bowl and drizzle some over the vinegar over it. Sprinkle with some sugar and stir as gently as you can to combine.

2. Grind some fresh pepper over it before serving.

CONCLUSION

I hope that with the conclusion of this book you are able to discover the wonder that Mediterranean cuisine has the potential to hold. This style of cuisine cannot only help you achieve whatever weight loss goals you may have, but it can also help you to live a much healthier lifestyle in the long run. Many people all over the world have adopted a mediterranean diet and lifestyle to boost their overall health and live much longer lives.

This guide is short in nature to simplify the concept. You can certainly build upon what you've learned here, and take the recipes, the concepts, and cater them to your individual needs and desires. For many, it is as simple as only keeping certain foods in their household to begin and continue the mediterranean lifestyle, and for others, it's a major paradigm shift to change their entire way of looking at their daily menu of options. We hope this guide gets you started and moving in the right direction to begin a better way of living.

PART 2

INTRODUCTION

I want to thank you and congratulate you for downloading the book, "Mediterranean Diet: Recipes and Diet Guide for Weight Loss and Healthy Eating".

This book contains proven steps and strategies to get to know more about the Mediterranean diet. This diet is considered to be the healthiest in the world. It is because it mainly calls for the consumption of vegetables, fruit, legumes, nuts, and unrefined cereals. When it comes to protein, you can never go wrong with seafood. Poultry and meats would have to take a back seat when you are in the Mediterranean diet though, and dairy products should be consumed in moderation. That good old wine can still be part of a good meal every once in a while.

In this book, you will know the health benefits of the Mediterranean Diet, the food pyramid, the Mediterranean Ingredients, how to choose olive oil and other Mediterranean recipes that you can easily follow at home. There are plenty of Mediterranean-inspired dishes to try and each one calls for ingredients that are easily found on your farmer's market or even at the grocery store.

Thanks again for downloading this book, I hope you enjoy it!

CHAPTER 1 ALL ABOUT THE MEDITERRANEAN DIET

THE MEDITERRANEAN DIET AND LIFESTYLE

This diet is a simple gastronomy with peasant origins. It is because the food that consist this diet is never pretentious as it is based with fresh fruits and vegetables, olive oil, beans and legumes, and with minimal animal protein and fat.

In the early 1990s, international nutritionists and scientists conducted a research on life expectancy in the

Mediterranean region and they have discovered that people living in the Mediterranean - the Spaniards, Greeks, and Italians among others - have lower incidence of cancer and heart diseases. It is surprising to note that their life expectancy is longer than those living in northern and central European nations and the United States. According to them, the Mediterranean diet coupled with low moderate intake of wine can contribute greatly to lowering heart diseases and cancer.

The Mediterranean diet advocates the abundant use of olive oil as a prime use of healthy fat. It has been a choice in the Mediterranean regions for centuries now and has been considered as one of the reasons why there is low occurrence of heart disease among Mediterranean people. The olive oil is a monosaturated oil that helps in lowering artery clogging LDL cholesterol and at the same time aids in keeping valuable levels of protective HDL cholesterol. Olive oil is also rich in vitamin

E that aids in neutralizing the free radicals in the blood stream causing tumors to develop and damaging the cells.

Other essential components of the Mediterranean region's cuisines are legumes and beans. These two replace meat providing important levels of protein, fiber, and complex carbohydrates.

It is also believed that the Mediterranean's rural lifestyle contributes to a stress-free living. The inhabitants of the Mediterranean consider their meals as a shared experience, usually in the company of family and friends. Taken communally, the Mediterranean diet is more than just food cooking and preparation – it has become their way of life.

WHAT CONSISTS THE MEDITERRANEAN DIET?

The best way to describe this diet is its focus on being physically active with the surrounding and the company of people are as important as the food. It may sound bizarre, but that is what the Mediterranean Diet Pyramid is all about.

Of equal value to social relationships and physical activity is the frequent consumption of fruits, vegetables, legumes, beans, whole grains, seeds, nuts, herbs, spices, and olive oil. If you are going to embrace this kind of diet, you have to be prepared in making these food a part of your every meal.

Each time a meal is planned and prepared, vegetables should be on top of the priority. It is for the reason that you will be filling half of your plate with these veggies either grilled, raw, steamed, boiled, or roasted. Also, they must be cooked to your enjoyment and with an abundance of natural herbs and spices.

The third most important part of the Mediterranean diet is seafood, which should be served for at least twice or thrice a week. Wild caught ones are recommended but it does not necessarily mean that they should be local to the Mediterranean region. What matters is that they are fresh and packed of natural nutrients.

CHAPTER 2 THE MEDITERRANEAN DIET FOOD PYRAMID AND HEALTH BENEFITS

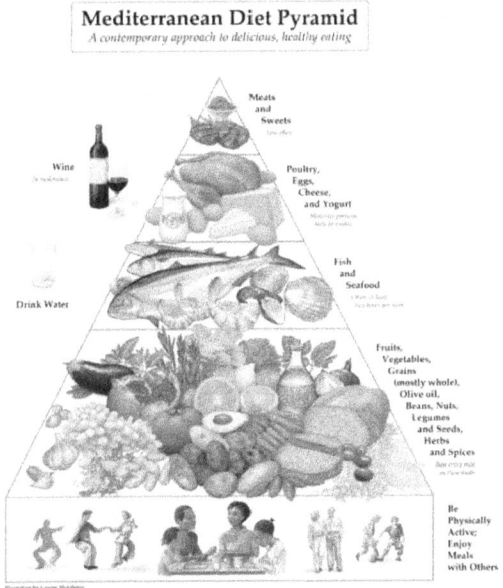

© 2009 Oldways Preservation and Exchange Trust • www.oldwayspt.org

According to research, the Mediterranean Diet Pyramid was developed and introduced by the World Health Organization, Oldways Preservation and Exchange Trust, a nonprofit educational organization, and the Harvard

School of Public Health. According to them, more than half of the area of the pyramid is made up of plant-based food illustrating the fact that meats are not the center of the plate, and are therefore marginal and must be consumed sporadically.

THE HEALTH BENEFITS OF THE MEDITERRANEAN DIET

Following the Mediterranean diet has abundant of health benefits to the body. You already know that this diet is consists mainly of fruits and vegetables, seafood, and olive oil among others. All these are main factors in keeping coronary heart diseases at bay as well as other hosts of health complications. On top of all these, you will notice that your body becomes healthier and stronger as you make the Mediterranean diet a lifestyle.

Here are the other health benefits that you will reap if you make a commitment to following the Mediterranean diet and lifestyle:

The risk of cardiovascular disease is lessened

Refined grains and sugar, red meat, and processed food are all linked to developing heart diseases and stroke. The Mediterranean diet discourages the consumption of all these so you will have lesser chances of having clogged arteries that could lead to heart diseases. Apart from this, this diet encourages drinking of red wine. So instead of going for the hard liquor, switch to a healthier version, something that is good for the heart. Just make sure not to go beyond the recommended intake of one drink for women and 2 drinks for men in a day or at least 5 ounces.

The chance of having type 2 diabetes is lowered

Did you know that eating processed food all the time could trigger high blood sugar that could eventually lead to diabetes? Following the Mediterranean diet helps reverse this and instead give the body gradual yet steady energy without the worries of your blood sugar going up the roof.

You get to lose weight the healthy way

Instead of following other fad diets that could either make you feel sluggish or deprived of necessary vitamins and nutrients, the Mediterranean diet helps you to naturally lose weight as it burns excess fat the moment you transition from eating high calorie, low nutrient food to abundantly nutritious, low calorie meals. This will make it easier for you to achieve your ideal body weight and figure out more ways to maintain it such as exercising, something that is considered a vital part of the Mediterranean lifestyle.

There is a reduced chances of being at risk of Parkinson's disease

The Mediterranean diet and lifestyle is high in antioxidants, which means that every cell in your body is abundantly supplied with the right kind of nutrients needed to shield you from oxidative stress considered to be one of the main reasons why people are at risks of said disease.

You become healthier - more strength and endurance

This is for as long as you follow the Mediterranean diet and lifestyle. One of the most attractive health benefits is the slowing down of aging and naturally boosting the body's physical capabilities.

With all said benefits, it is also important that you enjoy this lifestyle just as those from the Mediterranean regions for it to become a permanent part of your lifestyle, something that should be second nature to you.

CHAPTER 3 MEDITERRANEAN REGIONAL INGREDIENTS

The Mediterranean region is made up of 15 countries in 3 continents, all bordering on or influenced by the Mediterranean Sea. Said areas are blessed with fertile lands that are perfect for growing fruits, vegetables, herbs and spices, making the diverse Mediterranean cuisines known all over the world. This rich culinary heritage originated from the sea giving its name to the region.

The following are some of the most outstanding ingredients that make up the Mediterranean diet and cuisine:

- Capers – these are the flower bud of a bush that is native to the Mediterranean. The buds are either sun-dried, picked, packed in salt, or pickled in vinegar brine. Although capers are already cultivated, you will still see bushes in remote eras in the Mediterranean region. They have pungent yet distinct flavor that can be added to dishes in small amounts.

- Artichokes – this exemplary Mediterranean vegetable is visible throughout different Mediterranean cuisines. When purchasing artichokes, one of the things to know if they are still fresh is they should make a squeaky sound when touched and must be firm when squeezed. Check for worm holes and the shade of green should range from soft green color to olive green.

- Dried beans and legumes – These have been the main sources of protein in the Mediterranean region. They are used in soups and stews and are also used to make dips and spreads. When going to use for cooking, make sure you wash them on a colander with cold water and pick up foreign particles such as small pebbles. Also, there is no need to pre-soak beans overnight since they are easy to cook especially in the pressure cooker. Tip: do not add salt at the beginning of the cooking process as this will only harden the beans and legumes. You may do so towards the end or along with other ingredients.

- Eggplant – this vegetable is native of India and is combined with other vegetables from the Mediterranean region to be roasted, pickled, or sautéed.

- Cereals and grains – this is considered to be a vital part in the Mediterranean diet because these are high in complex carbohydrates. It should come as no surprise as Italians are the largest consumers of pasta in the world. Same goes with the people of Spain and Portugal enjoying food such as gachas and papas de milho. Grain is another key ingredient that Spaniards cannot go without. As they say, "Es mas largo que un dia sin pan" (It is as long as a day without bread). Finally, there is rice – the short grain variety of the region. Some of the best known short-grained rice in the region are Italian Arborio.

- Dairy – this is not that prevalent in the Mediterranean diet due to the absence of lands for cows, but milk-based products are made from goats or sheep's milk, both of which are available since the animals do not require large pastures. Cow's milk and butter are consumed in small quantities. Cheese, on the other hand, is more prevalent. Chesses like Parmesan and Pecorino Romano are mostly used as ingredients.

- Eggs – this is one of the vital sources of the Mediterranean diet that is not only consumed as part of their breakfast lifestyle but lunch and dinner as well.

- Fish and shellfish – this is enjoyed throughout the Mediterranean region. Some of them include cod, mackerel, tuna, squid, octopus, mussels, and shrimp among others.

- Meat and Poultry – these food are eaten in smaller quantities in the Mediterranean diet. This is not the main focus of the meal and are rather used to flavor dishes or accompany other components of a Mediterranean dish.

- Herbs and spices – the flavorings that are used in Mediterranean cooking are either introduced during the Middle Ages by natives to the area. Herbs such as parsley, oregano, thyme, cilantro, sage, and mint are just some of the herbs considered important in seasoning regional dishes.

- Garlic and onions – Mediterranean cooks adore the use of garlic and onions in their recipes. They even consider these two as the backbone of many delectable recipes of the region. The cloves of garlic, especially when unpeeled gives out a less forceful flavor, while onions add mellow sweetness to a dish. Indeed, no dish in this region is complete without these two.

- Potatoes – these are introduced to the Mediterranean region as a cheap source of nutrition for the natives. Today, potatoes are enjoyed throughout the region and are served in various ways such as fried in olive oil, as accompaniment to meat, boiled, and even as main ingredient for salads and soups.

- Peppers – this flavoring agent can either be fried, baked, or roasted. There are two types of peppers used in the Mediterranean cooking, the Italian peppers and the bell peppers. Both of which bring great flavor to Mediterranean dishes.

- Tomatoes – did you know that tomatoes were considered poisonous during the sixteenth century? It was not until the 19th century when it was finally accepted and became one of the most important ingredients in the Mediterranean cooking. Tomatoes are in their best flavor when vine-ripened and in season.

- Olive oil – this is perhaps the most important in traditional Mediterranean cooking. Olive oil plays a key role in maintaining a healthy diet for the people in the Mediterranean. This is cholesterol-free and help eliminate cholesterol from the blood by carrying it to the liver. There are many olive trees found in the region and the conditions under which they grow have a huge impact in the quality and flavor of the oil.

Olive oil is also said to be the chief source of fat in the traditional Mediterranean cuisine. During the ancient times, it is believed that the Arabs were the first ones to cultivate olive trees. Afterwards, planting olive trees spread throughout the region and the olive tree has long been held in high regard.

In the market, there are basically three retail grades of olive oil. The most expensive is the extra virgin olive oil that is obtained from the fruit of the olive tree only by physical or mechanical means. To be classified as extra virgin, the oil must be from the first cold pressing of the olives and an acidity level of no more than one percent.

Virgin olive oil can also be from the first cold pressing but can have an acidity level of 1.0 to 3.3 percent.

Finally, olive oil, considered to be the least expensive is a blend that is heat and chemically refined olive oil and virgin olive oil with an acidity level of less than 1.5 percent.

CHAPTER 4 MEAL PLANS AND RECIPES

BREAKFAST RECIPES

1. Berries and Mint Salad

Ingredients:

- 2 mint leaves, julienned
- ¼ lb fresh strawberries
- ½ cup fresh cranberries
- ½ cup fresh blueberries
- ½ cup fresh raspberries
- 1 teaspoon lime juice, freshly squeezed
- ½ teaspoon maple syrup

Directions:

1. Combine mint leaves, strawberries, cranberries, blueberries, and raspberries in a salad bowl. Toss well.
2. Place equal portions into salad bowls. Drizzle in lime juice and maple syrup on top. Serve immediately.

2. Green and Red Fruits with Walnut Salad

Ingredients:

- 8 green grapes, quartered
- 2 red apples, diced
- ¼ cup roasted walnuts, store-bought, lightly salted

For the Dressing

- 1 teaspoon extra virgin olive oil
- 3 teaspoon apple cider vinegar
- 1 teaspoon palm sugar, crumbled
- Pinch of kosher salt
- Pinch of white pepper

Directions:

1. Combine extra virgin olive oil, apple cider vinegar, palm sugar, salt, and pepper in a bottle with tight fitting lid.
2. Seal and shake bottle until ingredients dissolve. Mix green grapes, red apples, and walnuts in a bowl. Drizzle in dressing. Toss well to combine. Place equal portions into salad bowls. Serve.

3. Broccoli with Maple Syrup and Apple Cider Vinegar

Ingredients:

- 1/3 cup water
- 5 cups broccoli florets
- 1 teaspoon olive oil
- 1 tablespoon apple cider vinegar
- 1 tablespoon maple syrup
- Pinch pepper
- ¼ cup pumpkin seeds

Directions:

1. In a skillet, bring water to a boil. Stir in broccoli. Cook, covered for 3 minutes. Cook, uncovered, for another 3 minutes or until the water begins to evaporate and the broccoli tender.

2. Pour olive oil into the skillet. Stir for 2 minutes. Remove from heat.
3. Drizzle the broccoli with vinegar and maple syrup. Sprinkle with red pepper and salt. Top with pumpkin seeds.

4. Zucchini Salad Bruschetta

Ingredients:

- 1 wheat bread
- 1½ tablespoons spicy hummus

For the toppings:

- ½ tablespoon tomato, diced
- ½ tablespoon cucumber, diced
- ¼ tablespoon chives, minced
- ½ tablespoon pomegranate seeds
- Pinch of kosher salt
- Pinch of white pepper

Directions:

1. Spread hummus on bread. Heat in an oven toaster for 1 minute or until warmed through.
2. Combine tomato, cucumber, chives, and pomegranate seeds in a bowl. Season with salt and pepper. Spread mixture on top of bruschetta. Serve.

5. Spinach, Tomato, and Tofutti Cheese Frittata

Ingredients:

For the frittata

- 1 tablespoon olive oil
- 1 small onion, sliced
- 1 clove garlic, minced
- 1 package spinach
- 1/3 cup coconut milk
- 1 cup applesauce

- ½ cup Tofutti cheese

For the Salsa

- 1 tablespoon lime juice
- 2 green onions, minced
- 1 clove garlic, minced
- 4 tomatoes, chopped
- 2 tablespoons fresh cilantro, minced
- ¼ teaspoon salt
- 1/8 teaspoon pepper

Directions:

1. To make the frittata, preheat the oven to 350 F. In a skillet, pour oil. Swirl to coat.
2. Cook onion and garlic. Saute for 3 minutes or until translucent and fragrant. Tip in spinach.

3. Meanwhile, pour milk and applesauce in a bowl. Whisk until frothy.

4. Pour applesauce mixture over spinach. Cook for 7 minutes. Sprinkle cheese. Bake for 10 minutes.

5. To make the salsa: combine onions, garlic, tomatoes, cilantro, salt, and pepper in a bowl. Pour over frittata. Serve.

LUNCH RECIPES

1. Quick and Easy Vegan Pesto Pasta

Ingredients:

- 1 cup vegetable noodle of choice
- 2 tablespoons pesto sauce
- 1 tablespoon vegan cheese of choice
- Pinch of kosher salt
- extra virgin olive oil

Directions:

1. Combine vegan noodles, pesto sauce, and vegan cheese in a bowl. Season with salt.
2. Drizzle more olive oil if needed. Serve.

2. Spinach and Grape Tomatoes Salad

Ingredients:

- 2 teaspoons vegetable oil
- 4 teaspoons balsamic vinegar
- Dash of Worcestershire sauce
- ½ teaspoons sugar
- 3 cups loosely packed spinach
- ½ cup grape tomatoes
- 1 ounce Tofutti cheese

Directions:

1. Combine oil, vinegar, Worcestershire sauce, and sugar in a bowl, Mix well. Set aside.
2. Put spinach in a bowl. Tip in spinach and grape tomatoes.
3. Pour dressing onto the veggies. Top with cheese. Serve.

3. Coconut Curry Soup

Ingredients:

- 3 cups vegetable stock
- 1 shallot, quartered
- 1 garlic clove, chopped
- 1 thumb-sized ginger, grated
- 1 potato, diced
- 1 cup frozen coconut meat, unthawed
- 1 carrot, diced
- 1 tablespoon garam masala
- Pinch of kosher salt
- 1 can coconut cream, divided

Directions:

1. Pour all ingredients in a Dutch oven set over high heat except for the coconut cream. Stir. Bring to a boil.
2. Secure the lid. Turn down heat to lowest setting. Allow to simmer for 30 minutes. Turn off the heat. Tip in coconut cream. Adjust seasoning, if needed.
3. Ladle equal portion into bowls. Serve.

4. Asparagus Rice

Ingredients:

- 3 cups brown rice, cooked
- ½ lb thick-stemmed asparagus
- Pinch of kosher salt
- Pinch of black pepper
- 2 cups vegetable stock
- ¼ cup fresh parsley, minced

Directions:

1. Pour brown rice, asparagus, salt, and pepper in a rice cooker. Pour the stock. Stir well Secure the lid. Press cook.
2. Wait for the rice cooker to automatically shift to warm. Turn off the heat. Ladle recommended serving portions into bowls. Garnish with fresh parsley on top.

5. Baked Brussels Sprouts

Ingredients:

- Nonstick cooking spray
- 1 lb brussels sprouts
- ½ yellow onion, finely chopped
- 1 tablespoon olive oil
- ½ teaspoon ground black pepper

Directions:

1. Preheat the oven to 425 F. Pour cooking oil onto the baking sheet. Put a

steamer basket in a large pot and pour water. Bring to a boil.

2. Place the brussels in the steamer basket. Steam for 5 minutes. Remove brussels from the pot. Drain. Transfer to a bowl. Stir in onion, olive oil, and pepper.
3. Layer vegetables and bake for 15 minutes. Do not overcook. Serve.

6. Spinach-Stuffed Mushrooms

Ingredients:

- ½ cup water
- 1 package spinach, chopped
- 1/8 teaspoon salt
- 8 large mushrooms
- 1 tablespoon extra-virgin olive oil

Directions

1. Add water in a saucepan. Bring to a boil. Tip in spinach. Season with salt.
2. Meanwhile, Heat the olive oil in a skillet. Saute chopped mushrooms for 3 minutes or until golden brown. Remove from pan.
3. Add and sauté mushroom caps for 5 minutes. Transfer to a dish.
4. Drain spinach. Tip in sautéed mushrooms. Spoon the spinach mixture. Serve.

7. Mussels with Tomato Sauce

Ingredients:

- 1 tablespoon extra-virgin olive oil
- 1 onion, finely chopped
- 1 garlic clove, minced

- 1 stalk lemongrass, chopped
- 1 teaspoon whole coriander seeds
- 1 cinnamon stick
- Pinch of sea salt
- Pinch of peppercorns
- 1 can tomatoes with juice
- 2 cups fish stock
- 3 lbs mussels

Directions:

1. Heat the olive oil in a pan. Saute onions for 2 minutes.
2. Tip in garlic, lemongrass, coriander seeds, cinnamon stick, salt, and pepper. Cook for 4 minutes. Pour tomatoes with juice and fish stock. Bring to a boil.
3. Add mussels. Cover and cook for 20 more minutes. Discard mussels that did not open. Ladle into bowls. Serve.

Dinner Recipes

1. Stir-Fry Mixed Vegetables

Ingredients:

- 3 tablespoons vegetable oil
- 1 package containing frozen green vegetables
- 2 tablespoons water
- 2 tablespoons soy sauce
- 1 package fresh spinach

Directions:

1. Heat olive oil in a skillet. Add frozen vegetables. Stir fry for 5 minutes or until all vegetables are tender. Add water and soy sauce. Allow to simmer for 3 minutes. Tip in spinach.

2. Cover and let it steam for 3 minutes. Stir vegetables and cook for another 2 minutes.

3. Spoon liquid into bowl. Pour in vegetables. Serve.

2. Baked Tomatoes

Ingredients:

- ¼ cup fresh herbs (marjoram, parsley, and basil)
- 3 tablespoons extra virgin olive oil
- 2 cloves garlic, minced
- 3 large tomatoes, cut in half
- ½ cup grated bread crumbs
- ½ cup Tofutti cheese
- Pinch of salt
- Pinch of pepper

Directions:

1. Preheat the oven to 350 F.

2. Layer tomatoes in a baking dish. Combine extra virgin olive oil, herbs, garlic, tomatoes, bread crumbs, Tofutti cheese, salt, and pepper in a bowl. Mix well.

3. Sprinkle each tomatoes with equal portion of the mixture. Bake for 30 minutes. Serve.

3. Squash Soup

Ingredients:

- 1 tablespoon olive oil
- 1 garlic cloves, minced
- 1 white onion, mince
- 4 cups mushroom stock
- 1 butternut squash, cubed
- Pinch of kosher salt
- Pinch of white pepper
- ¼ cup cashew cheese
- ¼ cup fresh parsley, minced

Directions:

1. Pour olive oil into saucepan set over medium heat.
2. Sauté garlic and onion until tender and fragrant. Tip in mushroom stock, squash, salt, and pepper. Stir well. Bring to a boil.
3. Secure lid. Turn down heat. Allow to simmer for 30 minutes. Turn off heat. Cool before processing in a blender.
4. Adjust seasoning. Ladle into bowls. Garnish with cheese and parsley.

4. Corn and Spinach Rice

Ingredients:

- 2 cups brown rice
- 1 can coconut cream
- 1 cauliflower, sliced into bite-sized florets
- 1 carrot, diced
- 1 onion, minced
- 1 garlic clove, minced
- 1 tablespoon curry powder
- 1 teaspoon ginger, grated
- Pinch of kosher salt
- 2 cups vegetable stock

Directions:

1. Pour brown rice, coconut cream, cauliflower, coconut, onion, garlic, curry powder, ginger, and salt in a rice cooker. Pour the stock. Stir well.
2. Secure the lid. Press cook. Wait for the rice cooker to automatically shift to warm. Turn off heat. Serve.

5. Broccoli Noodles

Ingredients:

- 2 fresh broccoli stems
- Pinch of kosher salt

Directions:

1. Make deep scores on one side of broccoli stem. Scrape cut side of vegetable using a vegetable peeler. Repeat until you have a pile of noodles.
2. Place vegetables into a colander. Sprinkle salt. Toss well to combine.
3. Let vegetables "sweat". Drain and shake off excess moisture.
4. Layer broccoli noodles on a towel. Roll tightly. Do not rinse. Use as needed.

6. Zucchini Noodles

Ingredients:

- 2 zucchini
- Pinch of kosher salt

Directions:

1. Scrape cut side of zucchini using a vegetable peeler. Repeat until you have a pile of noodles.
2. Place vegetable noodles into a colander. Sprinkle salt. Toss well to combine.
3. Let vegetable "sweat". Drain and shake off excess moisture.
4. Layer zucchini noodles on a towel. Roll tightly. Do not rinse. Use as needed.

7. Carrot Noodles

Ingredients:

- 2 carrots
- Pinch of kosher salt

Directions:

1. Scrape cut side of carrots using a vegetable peeler. Repeat until you have a pile of noodles.
2. Place vegetable noodles into a colander. Sprinkle salt. Toss well to combine.
3. Let vegetable "sweat". Drain and shake off excess moisture.
4. Layer carrot noodles on a towel. Roll tightly. Do not rinse. Use as needed.

8. Fish Stew with Tomatoes and Anchovies

Ingredients:

- 1 tablespoon extra-virgin olive oil
- 2 onions, finely chopped
- 3 cloves garlic, minced
- 1 bulb fennel, diced
- 2 teaspoons dried Italian seasoning
- 1 teaspoon sea salt
- 1 teaspoon peppercorns

- 1 can diced tomatoes with juice
- 2 cups fish stock
- 1 ½ lbs firm white fish such as halibut
- ½ cup black olives, chopped
- 1 jalapeño pepper, diced

Directions:

1. Heat the olive oil in a pan. Saute onions and garlic for 3 minutes. Stir in fennel, Italian seasoning, salt, and pepper. Saute for 3 minutes. Pour tomatoes with juice. Bring to a boil.
2. Pour the fish stock. Cover and cook for 1 hour. Add the fish, olives, and jalapeno pepper. Cook for another 15 minutes.
3. Ladle stew into soup bowls. Serve.

DESSERT

1. Blue Cheese and Red Onion Marmalade

Ingredients:

- 300ml almond milk
- 300 ml coconut whipping cream
- 2 cloves garlic
- 4 peppercorns
- 1 bay leaf
- 1 cup applesauce
- 2 cups vegetarian soft blue cheese
- 2 tablespoons vegetarian sweet white wine

For the marmalade:

- 1 tablespoon olive oil
- 2 red onions, thinly sliced
- 1 tablespoon sherry vinegar
- 2 tablespoons sugar

Directions:

1. Warm the almond milk and cream. Tip in garlic and peppercorns. Soak for 10 minutes. Pour appleasauce. Mix until well combined.

2. Return mixture to the pan. Stir until the sauce thickens. Add cheese and pour wine. Let cool.

3. Put mixture in a container. Freeze. Once partially frozen, beat mixture and return to the freezer. Repeat procedure for three times.

4. To make the marmalade, saute onion in a skillet for 3 minutes. Add vinegar and sugar. Mix well. Bring to a boil for 10 minutes. Store in a jar. Serve either hot or cold.

2. Spinach Flat Cakes

Ingredients:

- 3 cups fresh spinach leaves

- 3 servings flax eggs
- ½ teaspoon garlic powder
- ²/₃ cup rice flour, finely milled
- 1 tablespoon baking powder
- ¼ teaspoon kosher salt
- coconut oil

Directions:

1. Put spinach and flax eggs in a blender. Process until smooth.
2. Add garlic powder, rice flour, baking powder, salt, and coconut oil. Except Pulse until ingredients are well combined.
3. Grease pan set over low heat. Pour an equal amount of spinach batter into the pan. Cook until edges are set. Flip once.
4. Cook the other side. Transfer to a tea towel. Serve.

3. Broccoli Flat Cakes

Ingredients:

- 3 cups broccoli florets
- 3 servings flax eggs
- ½ teaspoon garlic powder
- ²/₃ cup rice flour, finely milled
- 1 tablespoon baking powder
- ¼ teaspoon kosher salt
- coconut oil

Directions:

1. Put broccoli florets and flax eggs in a blender. Process until smooth.
2. Add garlic powder, rice flour, baking powder, salt, and coconut oil. Except Pulse until ingredients are well combined.
3. Grease pan set over low heat. Pour an equal amount of broccoli batter into the pan. Cook until edges are set. Flip once.
4. Cook the other side. Transfer to a tea towel. Serve.

4. Carrot Flat Cakes

Ingredients:
- 3 carrots
- 3 servings flax eggs
- ½ teaspoon garlic powder
- $^2/_3$ cup rice flour, finely milled
- 1 tablespoon baking powder
- ¼ teaspoon kosher salt
- coconut oil

Directions:
1. Put carrots and flax eggs in a blender. Process until smooth.
2. Add garlic powder, rice flour, baking powder, salt, and coconut oil. Except Pulse until ingredients are well combined.
3. Grease pan set over low heat. Pour an equal amount of carrot batter into the pan. Cook until edges are set. Flip once.

4. Cook the other side. Transfer to a tea towel. Serve.

5. Cranberry and Cherries Puddings

Ingredients:

- 1 cup dried cranberries
- 1 cup dried cherries
- 1 cup dates
- 1 apple, chopped
- ½ teaspoon freshly ground nutmeg
- 1 orange, zest and juice
- ½ cup olive oil
- 2 tablespoons brown sugar
- 1/2 cup applesauce
- 2 tablespoons almond milk
- 1 teaspoon vanilla extract
- 75g self-rising flour

- 75g breadcrumbs
- 2 cups ground almonds

Directions:

1. Preheat the oven to 300 F. Grease a muffin tin.
2. Combine put the cranberries, cherries, dates, apple, nutmeg, orange juice and zest in a saucepan, Bring to a boil for 3 minutes. Set aside.
3. In a separate bowl, combine oil and sugar. Beat well. Add applesauce. Stir the remaining ingredients until well combined. Put equal portions between tins. Bake for 1 hour or until the pudding is firm to touch.
4. Remove and let cool for 10 minutes. Serve.

6. Apricots and Cherries Puddings

Ingredients:

- 1 cup apricots
- 1 cup dried cherries
- 1 cup dates
- 1 apple, chopped
- ½ teaspoon freshly ground nutmeg
- 1 orange, zest and juice
- ½ cup olive oil
- 2 tablespoons brown sugar
- ½ cup applesauce
- 2 tablespoons almond milk
- 1 teaspoon vanilla extract
- 75g self-rising flour
- 75g breadcrumbs
- 2 cups ground almonds

Directions:

1. Preheat the oven to 300 F. Grease a muffin tin.

2. Combine put the apricots, cherries, dates, apple, nutmeg, orange juice and zest in a saucepan, Bring to a boil for 3 minutes. Set aside.

3. In a separate bowl, combine oil and sugar. Beat well. Add applesauce. Stir the remaining ingredients until well combined. Put equal portions between tins. Bake for 1 hour or until the pudding is firm to touch.

4. Remove and let cool for 10 minutes. Serve.

7. Swiss Chard Flat Cakes

Ingredients:

- 3 handfuls Swiss chard leaves, torn
- ¼ cup cashew nuts, roasted
- 3 servings flax eggs
- ½ cup all-purpose flour
- coconut oil
- 1 tablespoon baking powder
- ¼ teaspoon kosher salt

Directions:

1. In a blender, put Pour Swiss chard leaves, flax eggs, and cashew nuts. Process until smooth. Add all-purpose flour, coconut oil, baking powder, and salt. Pulse until ingredients are well combined.
2. Grease a pan set over low heat. Pour an equal amount of batter into the pan. Cook until edges are set. Flip once. Cook the other side. Put in tea towel. Serve.

CONCLUSION

It is my sincere hope that you might have liked all the recipes which have been mentioned in the book and once again thank you for getting this book and experimenting with the recipes.

ABOUT THE AUTHOR

Betty Leblanc is born with the vision to promote *Intermittent fasting* among the masses. The author has written several research papers on the topic. He has served as an instructor promoting various cultural arts in University of San Francisco. He is currently living with his spouse in Texas.

www.ingramcontent.com/pod-product-compliance
Lightning Source LLC
LaVergne TN
LVHW011950070526
838202LV00054B/4870